Vegan Athlete's Cookbook

Recipes rich in protein

Author

Charles L. Holt

Contents

- Top Tips for Building Lean Muscle on A Vegan Diet
- Breakfast Recipes
- Tofu Crumble with Vegetables
- Banana Almond Cream Shake
- Vegan Breakfast Sandwich
- Maple Ginger Pancakes
- Vegan Breakfast Tacos With Mango Pineapple Salsa
- Lunch Recipes
- Creamy Asparagus And Pea Soup
- Roasted Teriyaki Mushrooms and Broccolini Soba Noodles
- Chickpea Sunflower Sandwich
- Vegan Baked Beans
- Gnocchi Alla Romana
- Dinner Recipe
- Butternut Squash and Tempeh Tacos
- Green Bean Casserole
- Vegan Mushroom Stroganoff.
- Dessert Recipes

- Oatmeal No-Bake Bites
- Peppermint Mocha Crumb Cake 57 Apple Crisp 59
- Top Tips for Building Lean Muscle on A Vegan Diet
- Eat real food

Whole unprocessed foods will help you stay leaner, because what yo u see is what you get. There are no hidden nasties. While meat- free alterna tives can be delicio us, there are often hidden sugars ancl fats that prevent us from leani ng up and absorbing nutrient s .

2 . Macros

Do yo u eat a good balance of carbs, fats and pro teins? To build lea n muscle we neecl ali three in uniso n for mainte nance, muscle growth and muscle recovery. Complex carb s like oats and sweet potatoes will nourish your nervous system and give you the energy you need

to lift. Fats like avocado and nut s keep your heart healthy as well as help ing to bala nce hormones. Proteins like chickpea s and le ntils help you feel fuller for longer and repair faster.

3. M icronutrients

Eat the rainbow! Fruits and vegetables have so many vitamins and minerals and they are low in calories, which means you can have more of them; which is great if yo u are trying to lean up. Vitamins A, B, C,

D, potassium, magnesium and iron will help boost your immune system and are extremely impo rtant if yo u want to train hard for results. The choice is endless so be b rave - from veggies Like broccoLi, carrots, spinach and beetroot to fruits lik e ban anas, which help rebalanceelectrolytes and prevent muscle cramping.

4. Varie ty

You will go far on your journey to build lean muscle if you aren't afraid to step o ut of your comfort zone. It's very hard to stick to a plate of beans, sweet potato and courgette every day, bu t if you change it up it wiLI remain exciting. Even that same meal can be made interesting by spiralising the courgette or blencling the beans into a dip or making sweet potato mash. Keep it fresh!

5. Calorie s

It' s dead simple - eat mo re!

To build muscle you bave to create a calorie surp lus - eating more calo ries than your body burns thro ug h d aily activ ities, workouts and normai p hysio logical processes.

J ust be smart with yo ur food choices and you will see and feel the benefits.

6. Water

3

65 percent of our body is made up of water, so keeping hydrated will help keep you at your full strength. Maint aining adeguate hydratio n levels will also reduce protein breakdown and help with protein synthesis, which will help you grow. It also helps to lubricate between the joints, which will help to prevent pain.

7. Feeding times

Always try to ea t regularly and not just one or two large meals per day. Eat every few hours so that yo ur body has the energy it needs to perform and function at its best. Pre and post worko ut meals are the most important times to eat if yo u're loo king to gain muscle, so that yo u can have the energy to smash a workout and then be able to reple nish the muscle glycoge n depleted during your workout.

8. Good quality protein powder and bars

Do your research! As vegans we tend to get excited when we see that magica! VE sign, but don' t settle. There are so many types of protein out ther e, fro m hemp to pea. Ideally, you wa nt to pick one that has the least amount of ingredients, flavourings and thickeners that can be bad for the gut. A shake or a bar is always handy to have on you for a quick snack or to boost up your protein levels on a particular day.

9. Mobility and flexibility

Th e more range you have, the more muscle you can engage; and the more muscle you work, the more calories you burn doing it. It's one thing having more muscle, but it's another thing entirely to be able to move around with it.

5

10. Creatine

As vegans, our natural creatine levels tend to be a little lower than non-vegans. Adding a little extra from a supple ment (in powder or tablet form) can be extremely beneficiai for increased strength, cognitive skills and managing glucose levels.

11. Food and fitness tracking

Be accountable! It's the best way to track if you're eating enough of the right foods or getting benefits from yo ur workouts, whether that be in muscle mass or an increase in the weights being lifted. This way you can make little ad justments if progress stops.

12. Lift heavy

Heavy weights will challenge you and ultimately change you. Using big compo und movements like squats and deadlifts will build strength and muscle faster.

13. Multi-directional movement

Our bodies move multi-direction ally, so why sho uldn't we train like this? Bending, turning, twisting, forwards, back, side-to-side is th e best way to strengthen out stabiliser muscles that help support the bigger muscles and jo ints.

7

14. HIIT

High In tensicy In terval Tr aining is the guickest way tO ge t leane r, fitter and faster in one go. If yo u want to get lea ner and stronger, this is for you. Get a timer app and pick a couple of exercises . Something like a run on the spot and a mountain climber, 20 seconds work, 10 second s rest, then repeat both eight times.

15. Breathe

It' s a great way to cut cortisol (stress hormone) levels. \lVhen the body is s tr esse d in fig ht or flig ht mode it is drained guickJy and clings onto reserves like fat, stopp ing yo u being as lean as yo u co uld be. Thi s is wben the body repairs and reco vers; mentally, p hysic ally and emotionally.

8

Breakfast Recipes

9

Tofu Crumble with Vegetables

YELD: 4 serving

INGREDIENTS

2 tablespoons ghee 1 pound mixed vegetables

1 pound firm tofu (organic)

1 /3 cup soy sauce

1 / 4 cup white sesame seeds 1 / 4 cup black sesame seeds

1 teaspoon toasted sesame oil basil leaves (Torn) DIRECTIONS

1. Carefu1ly drain tofu

2. \Vrap tofu in paper towels and press to remove the excess liquid

3. Fili a bowl with water and put on top of wrapped tofu to press the liquid out 4. Leave for 15 min 5. Remove press and paper towels from tofu

6. Crumble tofu with your hands into sma11 pieces 7. Heat the oil in the pan on medium 8. Add vegetables to a pan and coo k for 10 min on medium heat, stirring often 9. Add tofu to vegetables and mix togethe r 1O. Cook tofu and vegetables for 5 more minutes

11. Add soy sauce, sesame seeds

12. Mix and cook for 1 min

13. Remove from heat, transfer to a large bowl and add sesame oil and mix again

14. Garnish with basi! and serve.

Banana Almond Cream Shake

YELD: 1 serving

INGREDIENTS

½ scoop brown rice p rotein powder, vanilla

½ scoop(s) pea protein powder 1 banana

1/2 cup s kim milk 10 whole almonds 1 handful ice

DIRECTIONS

1. Mix ingredients together in a blender and enjo y!

2. Alternate op tio ns for skim milk: almond, soy, coconut, or cashew milk.

13

Vegan Breakfast Sandwich

INGREDIENTS For the tofu:

1 block (350g) extra-firm tofu, *pressed fora minimum of 30 minutes, then cut into 4 slices 2 tablespoo ns nutritional yeast

2 tablespoons olive oil

14

2 tablespoo ns soy sauce 2 tablespoo ns water

1 teaspoon liquid smo ke 1 teaspoon Sriracha, or other hot sauce (optional)

1/ 2 teaspoon garlic powder

For the vegan breakfast sandwich:

4 English muffin s, sLic e d in half and toasted (glut e n-free if preferred)

1 avocado, mashed

1 large tornato, sLic e d Vegan To ast Dipping Sauce DIRECTIONS

1. To prepare the tofu: mix the nutritional yeast, olive oil, soy sauce, water, liquid smoke, Sriracha, and garlic powder together in a large resealable bag or a sma!J casserole dish. Add the t0fu piec es and tu.rn them to coa t evenly. Let marinate for a minimum of 30 minut es but the lo nger the better. I like to store my to fu covered the fridge so that I have marinateci slices ready to go in the morning. They sho uld keep for about 1 week.

2. \Xf hen you are ready to coo k the tofu, beat a large ski!

Je t o r fr ying pan over mediu.m- high heat. \Xfhen hot add the tofu slices and any remaining marinade. Cook for about 5 minutes on each side unti! golden brown. The marinade wiJI get sticky and brown, so just push it onto the t0fu with a spatula as this wil.l add even more flavou.r.

3 . T o pre pare the vegan breakfast sandwic h: take 1/ 4 of the mashed avocado and

spread it on the bottom laye r of an E nglish muffin. Top the avocado with a slice o f to fu, add 1 - 2 to rnato slices, drizzle as much or as little Vegan Toast Dipping Sauce as you like, and then add the English muffin top. Repeat with the remaining ingredients to make 4 sandwiches. Enjo y hot. I like serving the remaining Vegan Toast Dipping Sauce on the side for dipping (if there is any le ft).

16

Pancakes with Maple & Ginger

INGREDIENTS: 2 SERVINGS YELD

2 PEOPLE (7 medium pancakes) 1 gallon of water

1 teaspoon of baking powder kosher salt (1/2 tsp.)

1 / 4 teaspoon ginger powder

17

1 / 4 teaspoon spice for pumpkin pie maple syrup, 1/3 cup

water, 3/4 cup

1 / 4 cup crystallized ginger slices, minced + 1 tablespoon crystallized ginger slices (plus a little extra for garnish)

DIRECTIONS

1. Combine the first five ingredients in a medium bowl and whisk to combine.

2. Toss the syrup and water into a small hole in the flour mixture. Stir a few times more, then add the chopped ginger and stir until everything is well combined. It's okay if there are flour splatters. Avoid overmixing the ingredients.

3. In a large frying pan, heat the oil on low. Using nonstick cooking spray, coat the inside of the pan. Pour in 1/ 4 cup of the batter once the pan is hot. Allow to cook until bubbles appear on the surface, then flip and coat with nonstick cooking spray. Allow to cook until everything is browned and done.

4. Add the remaining batter to the pan and repeat the process. About seven medium pancakes will be made from this recipe.

5. Serve hot, with a dollop of vegan butter, a drizzle of maple syrup, and chopped candied ginger on top.

18

Mango Pineapple Salsa for Vegan Breakfast Tacos

4 tacos (small) YELD

19

THE FILLING INGREDIENTS ARE:

12 of the black bean tofu scramble recipe To make the Mango Pineapple Salsa, combine all of the ingredients in a blender and puree until smooth.

1 tblsp shallot (diced)

2 tsp garlic, minced

1/J c an an an an an an a tomatoes, chopped

12 c. pineapple, diced

12 c. mango (diced) 12 lime juice, 1 tbsp cilantro

1 seeded and diced jalepeno pepper (optional, but recommended) to taste salt and pepper (heavy on the pepper)

4 small soft tor tillas or 2 large tor tillas for the tacos avocado

extra lime and cilantro for garnish cilantro-lime avocado dressing (optional) (optional) DIRECTIONS

1. Throw ali the ingredients for the salsa into a bowl and mL"X well. Season to taste with salt and pepper.

2. Cover with plastic wrap and set aside in the fi-idge while you prep the tofu scramble

3. When the tofu scramble is ready, heat the tortillas in a skillet over medium heat for about a minute on each side.

4. Toss tofu scramble, avocados, mango pineapple salsa, extra lime juice, and cilantro-lime avocado dressing onto a plate (if desired)

Recipes for lunch

22

Soup with Asparagus and Peas (creamy Asparagus and Peas)

4 servings YELD: SOUP CONTAINS THE FOLLOWING INGREDIENTS

2 tablespoons oil (olive or avocado)

12 oz. asparagus (trimmed / 1 large bundle young s - 12 oz.)

eld - 10 ounces) fresh or frozen peas, 20 ounces (2 cups)

Garlic, 4 cloves (minced)

shallot (medium) (thinly sliced) seasoned with salt and pepper

1 and a half cup Almonds Breeze unsweetened unsweetened unsweetened unsweetened unsweetened unsweetened unsweetened unsweetened almond 1 1 and a half cup vegetable broth (DIY or store-bo ught)

1-2 tablespoons nutritional yeast (optional/ for a cheesy flavor) 1 /2 medium lemon (optional / / juiced / / for freshness) CRO UTO NS GA.RLIC HERB (op tional)

2 cups cubed bread (any variety)

a quarter-cup of extra virgin olive oil (or other neutral o il)

14 teaspoon garlic powder, salt + pepper, dried oregano, and dried basil

DIRECTIONS

1. Preheat the oven to 400 degrees F (204 degrees C) and spread the asparagus out on a baking sheet that hasn't been greased. Drizzle with your preferred oil and season with salt and pepper to taste. Toss to evenly distribute the ingredients.

2. Roast for 15 minutes, then set aside in an airtight container. Reduce the heat to 325°F if you're making croutons at this point.

3. Preheat medium heat in a large saucepan or pot. When the pan is hot, add 2 tablespoons oil (amount as written in the original recipe / / adjust if the size of the batter changes) and the shallot and garlic. Season with salt and pepper to taste and toss to coat. Cook until fragrant and translucent, about 2-3 minutes. If garlic starts to brown, turn down the heat.

4. Season with salt and pepper after adding peas, vegetable broth, and half-and-half.

24

more.

5. Combine the soup and asparagus in a blender (reserve some for garnish if desired). Unti unti unti unti unti

untiuntiuntiuntiuntiuntiuntiuntiuntiuntiun Return to the pot and reduce to a low heat setting to keep it simmering.

6. Finally, whisk in the nutritional yeast. Continue to cook until the sauce has warmed up and is simmering, then turn off the heat.

7. Season to taste with more salt and pepper if desired. Remove the pan from the heat and stir in the juice of one lemon.

8. Lower the oven temperature to 325 degrees F if serving with croutons while the soup is simmering.

9. In a mixing bowl, put bread crumbs. Whisk together the oil and seasonings in a separate bowl, then pour over the bread crumbs and toss to coat. Add a pinch of garlic powder, salt, and pepper to taste. Re-toss.

1O. Bake for 15-20 minutes or until golden brown on a clean baking sheet (or the one you used earlier). To ensure even baking, flip/ stir at the ten-minute mark.

11. Garnish with vegan parmesan cheese, croutons, and a pinch of black pepper. Leftovers can be kept refrigerated for up to a few days, but they're best when they're fresh.

25

Broccolini Soba Noocles with Roasted Teriyaki Mushrooms

YELLOW: 4 SERVINGS INGREDIENTS: Mushrooms:

26

Butto n mushrooms, 3 x 8 oz. containers 1 tablespoon of extra-virgin olive oil for high-heat cooking

1 tbsp vinegar de riz honey, 2 tbsp.

2 tbsp soy sauce (gluten-free) or tamari 1 tablespoon ginger, grated

Vegetables with Soba Noodles:

1 buckwheat soba noodles package (gluten-free) 1 teaspoon of extra virgin olive oil

12 shallots (12 shallots) 2 garlic cloves, minced

2 broccolini bunches, cut off the ends and cut the stems in half lengthwise if the stems are thick. kale, cut into shreds (about 5 stalks)

SOBA & OODLES SAUCE:

14 cup soy sauce (gluten-free) or tamari olive oil, 2 tablespoons

1 tablespoon toasted sesame oil and the juice of 1 lemon honey, 1 tablespoon

1 tsp. sriracha chili sauce 1 tablespoon ginger, grated Toppings:

green onions, chopped hot peppers, ses ame seeds, chopped ses ame seeds, chopped ses ame seeds, chopped ses ame seeds, chopped ses ame seeds, chopped ses ame seeds, DIRECTIONS

1. Preheat the oven to 425°F and grease a baking sheet. Remove the stems from the mushrooms, wipe away any dirt with a paper towel, and cut each mushroom in half before placing them in a large mixing bowl. \ Toss together the ingredients for the mushroom glaze. In a mixing bowl, pour the glaze over the mushrooms and toss to coat evenly. Place the mushrooms on a baking sheet lined with parchment paper and bake for 15 minutes. Remove them from the pan and toss them around to make sure they cook evenly. 15 minutes more roasting time

2. In the meantime, prepare soba noodles according to package directions, and heat a large skillet over medium heat with a tablespoon of olive oil. Cook for 1 minute after adding the minced garlic and Ed's Hallot. Cook until the broccolini and kale are tender, seasoning with salt and pepper to taste. 5 minutes or until just tender

3. In a mixing bowl, combine the soba noodle sauce ingredients while the vegetables and noodles are cooking.

4. Pour the sauce over the broccolini and kale in the pan and stir until the vegetables and noodles are evenly coated.

5. Divide the noodJes and vegetables between bowls and top with the roasted mushroom. Sesame seeds, hot peppers, and green onions can be added as garnishes.

Sandwich with Chickpeas and Sunflower

INGREDIENTS: 2 (sandwiches) YELD: 2 YELD: 2 (sandwiches) YELD: 2 YELD:

Sandwich

chickpeas, 15 oz (rinsed and drained)

sunflower seeds, unsalted, roasted 14 cup (if salted , scale back on added salt) vegan mayonnaise, 3 tbsp (sub tahini fora more earthy, nutty f:lavor)

1/ 2 tsp di jo n or spicy mustard (if using tahini instead of mayo, use half as much mustard) (if using tahini instead of mayo, use half as much mustard) 1 Tb sp maple syrup (or sub agave or honey if not vegan) (or sub agave or honey if not vegan)

1/ 4 cup chopped red onion

2 Tbsp fresh dill* (finely ch opped) (finely ch opped)

1 healthy pinch each salt and pepper (t0 taste) (t0 taste)

4 pieces rustic bread (lightly to asted / / gluten-free for GF eaters)

Sliced avocado, onion, tornato, and or lettuce (optional / / for serving)

Garlic H erb Sauce Op tional

1/ 4 cup hummus

1/ 2 medium lemon, juiced (1 / 2 lemon yields - 1 Tbsp) 3/ 4 - 1 tsp dried diii*\s2 cloves garlic (minced) (minced)

Water or unsweetened almond milk (to thin) (to thin) Sea salt tO taste (optional / / I didn't need any) DIRECTIONS

1. Prepare garlic herb sauce and set aside.

2. Add chickpeas to a mixing bowl and lig htly mash with a fork for texture. Then add sunflower seeds, mayo, mustarcl, maple syrup, red onion, diii, salt, and pepper and

mix with a spoon. Taste and adjust seasonings as needed.

3. Toast bread (if desired) and prepare any o ther sandwich toppings you desire (tornato, onion, lettuce).

4. Scoop a healthy amount of filling onto two of the pieces of bread, add desired toppings and sauce, and top with o ther two slices of bread.

5. Sunflower-chickpea mixture will keep covered in the fridge for up to a few days, making it great for quick weekday lunch es!

NOTES *1 Tbsp dried diii can be subbed per 2 Tbsp fresh.

*2-3 tsp fresh dill ca n be subbed per 3/ 4-1 tsp dried.

31

Vegan Baked Beans

YELD: 6 serving

INGREDIENTS 1 tbsp. vegetable o il

32

1 large onion, sliced into thin strips 1 / 4 cup bourbon whiskey

2 garlic cloves, minced 1 /3 cup tornato paste

2 tbsp. vegan Worchestershire sauce 2 tbsp. blackstrap molasses

2 tbsp. apple cider vinegar 2 tbsp. soy sauce

1 tbsp. prepared mustard 1 tsp. smoked paprika

1 tsp. liquid smoke, optional

1/ 4 to 1/2 cup mapie syrup, see my note

2 (14 oz.) cans navy beans or great northern beans, drained and rinsed

salt and pepper to taste

DIRECTIONS

1. Coat the bottom of a skillet (use a medium, oven-safe skillet if you 've got o ne) with oil and piace over medium -low heat. Add onion and toss a few times to coat. Allow to cook, flipping occasionally, unti! onio n is very sof t and caramelized, 30-40 minutes. Raise heat to medium and add garlic. Cook unti! very fragrant, about 1 minute more. Add whiskey and bring to a simmer. Allow to cook unti! most of the liquid has cooked off, about 4 minutes. Remove from heat.

2. Preheat oven to 350°. Stir tornato paste, Worchestershire sauce, molasses, apple cider

vinegar, soy sauce, mustard, paprika and liquid smoke toge ther in a small b ow l. Stir in 1/ 4 cup mapie syrup, taste test and add up to 1/ 4 cup more. If you used a non ove n-safe skillet to caramelize the onions, transfer them to an oven-safe dish (an 8 inch x 8 inch baking dish works). Othe1wise, leave them in the oven-safe skillet. Add bea ns and maple sy rup mixture. Stir a few times to mix everyth ing up. Season with salt and pepper to taste.

3. Cover and bake 40-45 minutes, unti! bubbly. Uncove r and bake 10 minute s more.

4. Remove fro m oven and allow to sit for a few minutes. Serve.

Gnocchi Alla Romana

YELD: 4 - 6 Servings INGREDIENTS

1 quart (4 cups) 2 percent or whole milk

1 heaping cup (175 grams) semolina flo ur (not fast-coo king variety)

1 teaspoo n kosher salt, plus more as desired

4 tablespoo ns unsalted butter, divided, plus more for greasing

1 hea ping cup (3.5 ounces) freshly grated Parmigiano-Reggiano cbeese freshly gro und black pepper

2 large egg yolks

DIR ECTIONS

1. Heat the milk in a large saucepan over medium-high beat until tiny bubbles start to form around the edges of tbe pan and tbe liquid is just sbort of boilin g.

2. Reduce tbe beat to lo w and slowly add tbe semolina flo ur in a very tbin steady stream with one hand as yo u stir tbe mixture steadily with a stiff large wbisk. The mixt ure will cook for rougbly 15 to 20 minutes t0tal, or unti! it becomes very thick and begins tO pull away from tbe side s o f the pan. It will be very loose for the first few minutes and will tbicken to tbe consistency o f a loose pudding witbin about 5 minutes. Once tbe mixture thick enough that it becomes difficult to continue whisking, switch to a wooden spoon. Continue stirring witb a wooden spoon, scraping tbe sides of the pan as well, unti! the mixture begins tO form a loose-isb mass and begins to pull away from the sides (approximately 15 to 20 minut es of tota! coo k time). Remove from the hea t. Allow tbe mixture to cool for a minute or two.

3. Stir in 2/3 of the grated parmesan cheeses, 2 tablespoo ns unsalted b utter, and salt. Season to taste with salt and freshly ground pepper.

Allowin g the mixt ure to cool sligbtl y will also pre vent the eggs from coagulating. Add the egg yolks and mix

rapidly with a wooden spoon unti! fully incorporateci.

4. Moisten a half sheet pan with cold water over a sink and allow the excess water to drip off the pan. Spoo n the hot semolina mixture onto the moistened sheet pan, spreading it with an offset spatula into an even layer that is just under 1 / 2-inch thick. Let coo l for 30- 40 minutes.

5. Preheat the oven to 425 degrees with a rack in the center positio n. Grease the bo tto m and sides of an oven-safe baking clish (roughly 2 qu arts in capacity) with unsalted butter. Using a small biscuit cutter

(roughly 2.5 -inch), cut the semolina into disks, clippin g th e bi scuit cutter into water continuo usly to pr eve nt sticking. Tr ansfer and layer the semolina rounds into the greased baking dish, o verlapping the slices s.lig htl y with each row to resemble roof shingles. Di stribute the top of the pole nta with the remaining 2 tablespoo ns butter, divided into smalJ pieces. Sprinkle t he top with the remaining grated cheese . G nocc hi alla romana can be prepped ahead up this stage and stored, covered with plastic wrap, in the refrigerator for up to 2 days.

6. Bake uncovered at 425 for 15 to 20 minutes or unti! a lig ht golden crust is formed. AUo w to cool for a few minut es befo re serving.

37

Dinner Recipe

Butternut Squash and Tempeh Tacos

YELD: 10 tacos

INGREDIENTS For the tacos:

1 small butternut squash, peele d and cut in 1/ 2-inch cubes 4 tbsp olive oil, divided 1 tsp cumin 1 / 2 tsp cinnamo n 1 / 4 tsp salt

1/ 4 tsp pepper

1 / 2 medium yellow onion, chopped 2 cloves garlic, minced

1 1 / 2 tbsp taco seasoning Juice of 1/ 2 lim e 8oz package of tempeh, crumbled (using your hands)

1/ 2 small bunch of cilantro, stems removed and chopped

1O corn tortillas

Avocado slices and lime wedges to serve

Optiona1 top pings for vegetarians: queso fresco and/ or plain Greek yogurt

For the Salsa Verde (adapted from Confessions of a Foodie):

1/ 216 tom atillos, husks removed and rinsed

1 jalapefio pepper, cut in half length wise, veins removed

1 / 2 medium yellow onion (chop 1/ 4 onion and leave the other 1/ 4 whole)

1 d ove garlic

1/3 cup water

1/ 2 tsp lime juice

1 /4 tsp salt

1 /2 small bunch of cilantro, stems removed and chopped

DIRECTIONS For the tacos: 1. Toss the butternut squash with 2 tbsp olive oil, cu min, cinnamon, salt and pepper.

40

Piace squash on a large skillet ove r mectium-high heat and cook unti! tender and browned, abo ut 10-15 minutes.

2. In a la rge saucepan, add oli ve oiJ o ver medium heat. O nce oil is hot, add cho pped onion and cook for about 3 minutes. Add garLic, and let coo k for another couple minutes, unti! fragrant and before browning.

3. Add crumbled temp eh, taco seasoning, Lime juice, and stir to combine. Let cook for ano ther couple minutes, remove from heat and add cilantro.

4. Piace corn tortillas over an open flame (mectium beat) on the st◊ve top. Let cook until to rtilla begins tO bubble and brown, less than a minute. Using tongs, flip over tO cook the other side, unti!. it begi ns tO brown and bubble.

5. Assemble tacos by adding the tempeh mixture, butternut squ ash, and salsa verde. Top with a squeeze of lime and avocado slices.

6. O ptio nal for vegetarians: add queso fresco and/ or plain G ree k yogurt as a t◊ pping.

For the Salsa Verde (adapted fro m Confessio ns of a Foodie):

1. Roast tomatillos, o nion wedge, garlic, and jalape no on a Lig htly greased skillet o ver mectium-high heat. Using tongs, continue to rotate vegetables so that they're bLis t e red on every side. Roast unti! tender and bLis t ered, about 1O minute s (note: tomatillos will take lo nger).

2. Transfer onion, pepper, garLic, and tomatillos to a food processor. Add li me juice and water. Pulse tO combine unti! smooth. Add salt to taste. Transfer tO a serving bowl and stir in cho pped o nion and cila ntro .

NOTES Tomaòllos will take lo nger to roast (wait until they start to release their juices to remove from heat).

42

Socca Pizza

INGREDIENTS: 2 SERVINGS YELD

2 tbsp olive oil

1 cup chick pea flo ur 1 cup water

1/ 2 tsp garlic pow der 1 tsp mi.xed dried italian seasoning, basil, oregano etc.

43

Salt and pepper, to taste

Super easy pizza sauce:

1/ 2 cup tornato passata 2 tbsp tornato puree

1 / 2 red onion

3 garlic cloves

1 tb sp dried italian seasoning

Toppings:

Cashew cheese sauce Fresh chopped basi!

Chopped veggies of choice, I used red onion and pepper

DIRECTIONS

1. Preheat the oven to 230C / 450F and brush a 35x20cm / quarter sheet baking tray with one tablespoon of the oil. Alternatively, you can use a large, round pizza tray.

2. In a medium bowl, mix together the remaining one tablespoon of oil, chickpea flo ur, water and seasonings. Whisk unti! completely smoo th.

3. Pour the batte r onto the baking tray and tilt to make sure the tray is evenly coated . Cook for 10 minutes unti! golden and slightly crisp. Remove from the oven but keep the oven hot.

4. Meanwhile, make the pizza sauce by simply blending the ingredients in a blender unti! smoot h. Spread on top of the socca base.

5. Drizzle dollops of the cashew cheese over the sauce and scatter some chopped

vege tables o n top. Bake again for a further 5-10 minutes. If you prefer yo u can drizzle the cheese on after the pizza has baked, for a more creamy cheese.

6. Cut into 6 slices and en jo y!

45

Tacos Sin Carne

4 servings YELD:

INGREDIENTS

Tacos:

2 Thsp sesame oil (or othe r vegetab le o il) 2 lb s. cremini or Portobe Uo mushrooms 1 Thsp gro und cumin

1 Thsp chili powder

1/2 tsp chipotle powder V4 tsp salt

8 tortillas 4.5 inch (flour or glut en-free corn)

2 limes quartered

2 avocados sliced (optional)

Pico de gallo:

1 yellow onion or white 2 jalapefio peppers

11.2 bunch cilantro

1 tornato (preferably heirloom)

DIRECTIONS

1. Dice onion, ja lapefio s, tornato and cilantro and combine in a bowl and set aside. Your pico de gallo is clone! Wasn't that easy?!

2. Remove the stems from the mushrooms and slice into ¼" slices.

3. Heat the sesame oil in a pan on mediurn-high heat. Add the sliced mushrooms, curnin, chili, chip otle and salt and sauté unti! mushrooms are fully cooked, around 7- 10 minut es.

4. Serve seasoned, cooked mushroo ms in warmed tortillas and top with pico de gallo and avocado slices. Serve with quartered limes on the side- these add some tangy brightness to the spice!

47

Green Bean Casserole

YELD: 4 serving INGREDIENTS

48

1 pound green beans (rinsed, trimmed and cut in half) Sea salt and black pepper

2 Thsp vegan butter or olive oil 1 medium shallo t (minced)

2 cloves garlic (minced)

1 cup finely ch opped mushrooms (button, baby be lla, or cremini) 2 Th sp all-purp ose flo ur

3/ 4 cup vegetable br o th (DIY or store-bought) 1 cup unsweetened plain almo nd milk

1 1 / 2 cu ps crispy fried onions (divided / / I lo ve Trader's Brand - check ingredients to ensure vegan friendly)

DIRECTIONS

1. Preheat oven to 400 degrees F (204 q . Bring a large pot of water to a boil and salt well - it will help season the green beans. Add green beans and cook for 5 minutes, then drain and piace in an ice water bath to sto p coo king. Drain and set aside.

2. In the meantime, start preparing sauce. In a large oven-safe skille t o ver medium hea t, add vegan butter or olive oil and shallots and garlic. Seaso n with salt and pepper and stir. Coo k for 2-3 minutes,

then add mushro oms and season with a bit more salt and pepper. Cook for 3-4 minutes more or unti! lig htly browned.

3. Sprinkle in flour and whisk to stir and coat the veggies. Cook for 1 minute, then slow ly add in veggie stoc k, whisking to incorporate.

4. Add almond milk next and whisk to stir again. Seaso n with a touch more salt and

pepper and bring to a simmer, then reduce heat to low to thicken. Cook for 5-7 minutes more, or unti! thick and bubbly. Taste and adjust seasonings as needed.

5. Remove from heat and add 1/ 3 of the fried onions (1/ 2 cup as origina! recipe is written / / adjust if altering batch size) and all of the cooked green beans. Toss to coat well, and top with remaining fried onions.

6. Bake for 15 minutes, or unti1 warmed through and bubbly and slig htly bro wned on top. Serve immediately (handle pan carefully).

7. Leftove rs sto re well in the fridge for up to a few days.

50

Vegan Mushroom Stroganoff

4 servings YELD:

INGREDIENTS For the Vegan Mushroom Stroganoff:

3 Tb sp (45g) Vegan Butter 1 Onion (Finely Chopp ed)

51

1 Tbsp Crushed Garlic

18oz (500g) Button Mushrooms* 3 Tb sp Ali Purp ose Flour

2 cups (480ml) Vegetable Stock (Strained)* 1 Tbsp Dijon Mustard

1 Tbsp Soy Sauce

1 Full Batch Vegan Sour Cream

* Salt and Pepper (To Taste)

For Serving: 1 / 2 Pack (-9oz/250g) Pasta (Dry Weight)* Chopped Chives (For Serving) DIRECTIONS

1. Put the pasta on to cook according to the package instruc tions.

2. Get ali your ingredients ready for yo ur sauce.

3. Th en add in the vegan butter to a pot along with the chopped onions sauté unti! the onions are softened. Then add in the sliced mushrooms and crushed garlic and fry unti. I the mushroom s are softened.

4. Add in the flo ur and fry with the mushrooms and onions for 1 minute. Then add in the vegetable stock and stir in unti! combined. Add the soy sauce and dijo n mustard and then the full batch of vegan sour cream.

5. Simmer unti! thickened.

6. Serve over the pasta with some chopped chives.

NOTE: *We used brown button mushroo ms - also called portobellini mushrooms, baby bella mushrooms or cremini mushrooms. You can also use regular white button mushrooms in this recipe.

*

You o nly need to strain your vegetable stock if it has pieces of dehydra ted vegetables in it. *

If you are using a di fferent vegan sour cream and not making yo ur own, then the amount to use is 1 cup (8oz/ 226g). If yo u make yo ur own using our recipe, then just use ali of it in this recipe.

*

We used papardelle pasta in this recipe (wide flat pasta noodles), but you can use any pasta th at you like. *

If yo u'd like to make this meal glut en-fr ee th en serve it with gluten-free pasta and use 1 and 1 / 2 Tbsp cornstarch instead of ali purpose flo ur or a gluten-free ali purpose flour blend. Also make sure yo ur soy sauce is gluten-free or switch it for tamari instead.

Oatmeal No-Bake Bites

Yield: 24 bites INGREDIENTS

1 cup roUed oat s (or gluteo-free oats)

1 cup coconut powder (or toasted coconut flakes) (or toasted coconut flakes) 1 / 2 cup carob chips

1/ 2 cup peanut butter

1 / 2 cup ground flaxseed

1 /3 cup agave nectar or mapie syrup 1 teasp. vanilla extract

DIRECTIONS

1. In a mi,-xing bo wl, combine all of the dry ingredients.

2. Add the peanut butter, honey (or agave nectar), and vanilla extract and thoroughly\smix to combine ali the ingredients.

3. Let the mixture chili in the fridge for about 30 minutes.

4. Once they are chilled, roll them into 1" diameter bal1s (you can use a cookie scooper to do this step) (you can use a cookie scooper to do this step).

5. Store in an airtight container and keep refrigerated.

Peppermint Mocha Crumb Cake

Yield: 8 servings

INGREDIENTS

1 cup non-dairy milk

1 /3 cup vegan mayo nnaise 1 / 3 cup brewed coffee

1 tables poon white distilled vinegar

1 cup unbleached all-p urpose flo ur or whole wheat pastry flo ur 2 tablespoo ns stevia

1 teaspoon baking powder

1 teaspoo n baking sod a 1/ 4 cup cocoa powder

1 teaspoo n gro und cinnamo n\s1 / 4 teaspoo n salt

3/ 4 cup unbleached all-purp ose flour or whole whea t pastry flo ur 1 / 4 cup brown sugar

3/ 4 cup crushed peppermint candy 1 / 2 teaspoo n gro und cinn amon

1 / 4 tea spoon salt

1/ 3 cup vegan butter, melted\sDIRECTION S

6. Preh eat the o ven to 350° F. Lightly grease a 9-inch baking dish/ cake pan.

7. To make the cake, whisk the milk, vegan mayonn aise, coffee, and vinegar together in a bowl and set aside. In a large bowl, mi x to ge ther the flo ur, stevia, cocoa powder, baking powder, baking so d a, cinnamon, and salt. Add the milk mixture and stir unti! just comb ined. Pour into the prepared baking dish.

8. To make the crumble, in a small bowl, combine the flour, sugar, cinnamo n, ginger, salt, and peppermint. Add the melte d vegan butter and use your hands to tho ro ughly work it into the dry ingredient s. Spoon on top of the batter, covering the entire area.

9. Bake for 35-40 minute s, or unti! a toothpick inserted into the middJe co mes o ut clean. Let it cool slight!y, and serve warm or at room temperatu re.

58

Appie Crisp

Yield: 10 servings\sINGREDIENTS\sFilling

59

8 medium-large apples (4 tart (like g rann y smith), 4 sweet (like honey crisp) / organic when possible)

1 lemon, juiced (1 lemon yields - 2 Thsp or 30 ml) (1 lemon yields - 2 Thsp or 30 ml) 2/ 3 cup coconut sugar (or sub organic cane sugar) (or sub organic cane sugar) 1 1 / 2 tsp ground cinnamo n\s3 Thsp arrowroot starch or cornstarch (for thickening) (for thickening) 1 / 4 cup fresh apple juice (or water) (or water)

3/ 4 tsp fresh grated ginger (optional / / or sub 1/ 2 tsp ground ginger per 3/4 tsp fresh)

1 pinch nutmeg (optional) (optional)

Topping

1 cup gluten-free rolled oats

1/ 2 cup almon d meal

1 / 2 cup unbleached all-pur pose flour*

1 / 2 cup coconut sugar (or sub organic cane sugar) (or sub organic cane sugar)

1 /2 cup muscovado sugar (or sub organic brown sugar) (or sub organic brown sugar)

1/2 cup pecans (roughly chopped) (roughly chopped)

1/ 4 tsp sea salt

1 t sp ground cinnamon

1 / 2 cup melted coconut oil or olive oil (or mix the two 1/ 2, 1/ 2)

DIRECTIONS

1. Preheat oven to 350 degrees F (176 C) (176 C).

2. Peel apples, quarter, remove cores, and use a paring knife to thinly slice lengthwise

(see pho to).

3. Add to a large mixing bowl and top with remaining filling ingredients. Toss to combine. Add to a 9x13 (or similar size / / as originai recipe is written / use smaller or larger is altering batch size) baking dish.

4. Rinse and wipe out your mixing bowl and add all to pping ingredients. Stir to combine, then use fingers to break down any clumps of musco vado sugar. Pour over apples in an even layer.

5. Bake for 50 minutes to 1 hour (uncovered) or unti! the filling is bubbly, the apples are very fo rk tender (especially in the center of the dish), and the topping is deep golden brown.

6. Let rest at least 30 minutes before serving. This is delicio us with coconut whipped cream or vanilla bean cocon ut ice cream.

7. Best when fresh, th ough leftovers keep covered in the refrigerator up to 3 days, or in the freezer up to 1 month. Reheat in the microwave or in a 350-degree F (176 C) oven unti] warmed through.

6155

1 cup coconut powder (or toasted coconut flakes) (or toasted coconut flakes) 1 / 2 cup carob chips

1/ 2 cup peanut butter

1 / 2 cup ground flaxseed

1 /3 cup agave nectar or mapie syrup 1 teasp. vanilla extract
DIRECTIONS

1. In a mi,-xing bo wl, combine all of the dry ingredients.

2. Add the peanut butter, honey (or agave nectar), and vanilla extract and thoroughly\smix to combine ali the ingredients.

3. Let the mixture chili in the fridge for about 30 minutes.

4. Once they are chilled, roll them into 1" diameter bal1s (you can use a cookie scooper to do this step) (you can use a cookie scooper to do this step).

5. Store in an airtight container and keep refrigerated.

56

Peppermint Mocha Crumb Cake

Yield: 8 servings

INGREDIENTS

1 cup non-dairy milk

1 /3 cup vegan mayo nnaise 1 / 3 cup brewed coffee

1 tables poon white distilled vinegar

1 cup unbleached all-p urpose flo ur or whole wheat pastry flo ur 2 tablespoo ns stevia

1 teaspoon baking powder

1 teaspoo n baking sod a 1/ 4 cup cocoa powder

1 teaspoo n gro und cinnamo n\s1 / 4 teaspoo n salt

3/ 4 cup unbleached all-purp ose flour or whole whea t pastry flo ur 1 / 4 cup brown sugar

3/ 4 cup crushed peppermint candy 1 / 2 teaspoo n gro und cinn amon

1 / 4 tea spoon salt

1/ 3 cup vegan butter, melted\sDIRECTION S

6. Preh eat the o ven to 350° F. Lightly grease a 9-inch baking dish/ cake pan.

7. To make the cake, whisk the milk, vegan mayonn aise, coffee, and vinegar together in a bowl and set aside. In a large bowl, mi x to ge ther the flo ur, stevia, cocoa powder, baking powder, baking so d a, cinnamon, and salt. Add the milk mixture and stir unti! just comb ined. Pour into the prepared baking dish.

8. To make the crumble, in a small bowl, combine the flour, sugar, cinnamo n, ginger, salt, and peppermint. Add the melte d vegan butter and use your hands to tho ro ughly work it into the dry ingredient s. Spoon on top of the batter, covering the entire area.

9. Bake for 35-40 minute s, or unti! a toothpick inserted into the middJe co mes o ut clean. Let it cool slight!y, and serve warm or at room temperatu re.

58

Appie Crisp

Yield: 10 servings\sINGREDIENTS\sFilling

59

8 medium-large apples (4 tart (like g rann y smith), 4 sweet (like honey crisp) / organic when possible)

1 lemon, juiced (1 lemon yields - 2 Thsp or 30 ml) (1 lemon yields - 2 Thsp or 30 ml) 2/ 3 cup coconut sugar (or sub organic cane sugar) (or sub organic cane sugar) 1 1 / 2 tsp ground cinnamo n\s3 Thsp arrowroot starch or cornstarch (for thickening) (for thickening) 1 / 4 cup fresh apple juice (or water) (or water)

3/ 4 tsp fresh grated ginger (optional / / or sub 1/ 2 tsp ground ginger per 3/4 tsp fresh)

1 pinch nutmeg (optional) (optional)

Topping

1 cup gluten-free rolled oats

1/ 2 cup almon d meal

1 / 2 cup unbleached all-pur pose flour*

1 / 2 cup coconut sugar (or sub organic cane sugar) (or sub organic cane sugar)

1 /2 cup muscovado sugar (or sub organic brown sugar) (or sub organic brown sugar)

1/2 cup pecans (roughly chopped) (roughly chopped)

1/ 4 tsp sea salt

1 t sp ground cinnamon

1 / 2 cup melted coconut oil or olive oil (or mix the two 1/ 2, 1/ 2)

DIRECTIONS

1. Preheat oven to 350 degrees F (176 C) (176 C).

2. Peel apples, quarter, remove cores, and use a paring knife to thinly slice lengthwise

(see pho to).

3. Add to a large mixing bowl and top with remaining filling ingredients. Toss to combine. Add to a 9x13 (or similar size / / as originai recipe is written / use smaller or larger is altering batch size) baking dish.

4. Rinse and wipe out your mixing bowl and add all to pping ingredients. Stir to combine, then use fingers to break down any clumps of musco vado sugar. Pour over apples in an even layer.

5. Bake for 50 minutes to 1 hour (uncovered) or unti! the filling is bubbly, the apples are very fo rk tender (especially in the center of the dish), and the topping is deep golden brown.

6. Let rest at least 30 minutes before serving. This is delicio us with coconut whipped cream or vanilla bean cocon ut ice cream.

7. Best when fresh, th ough leftovers keep covered in the refrigerator up to 3 days, or in the freezer up to 1 month. Reheat in the microwave or in a 350-degree F (176 C) oven unti] warmed through.

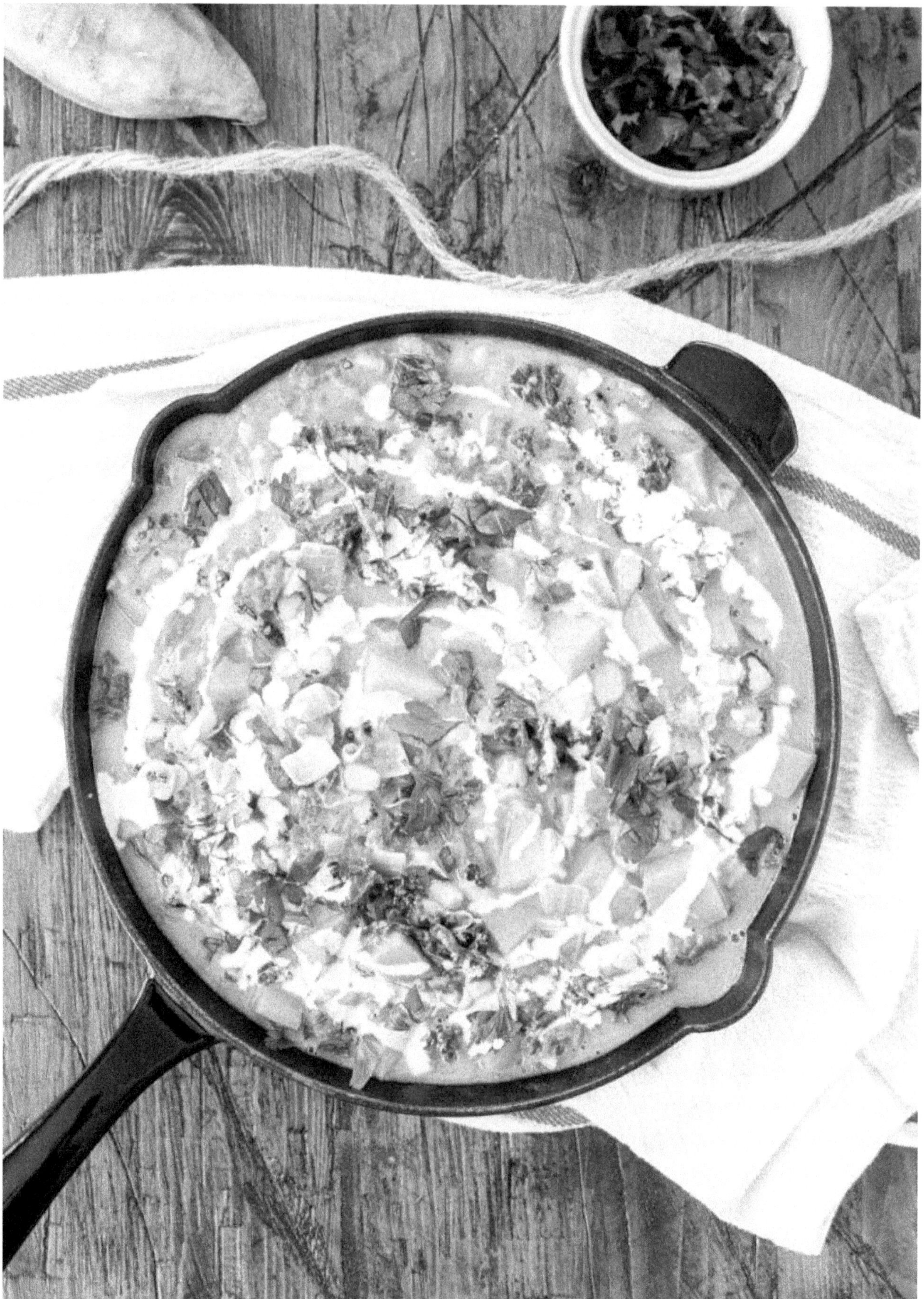

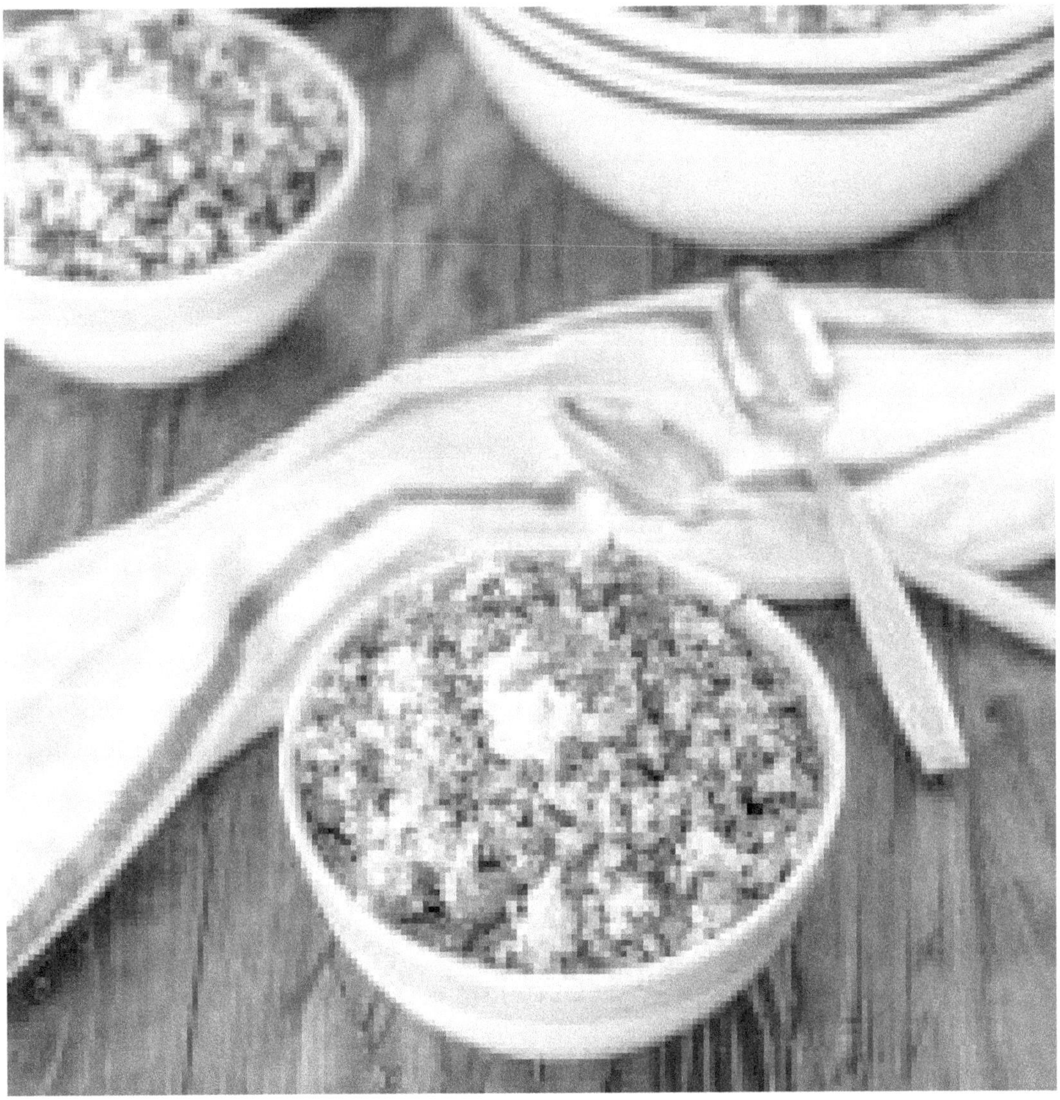

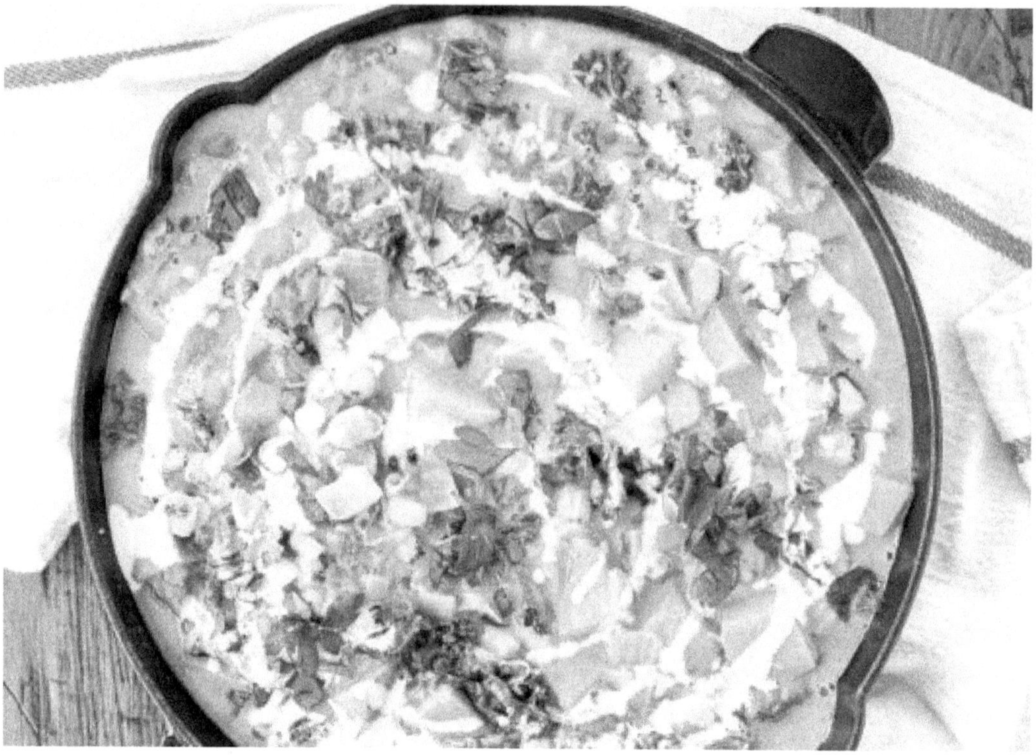

CPSIA information can be obtained
at www.ICGtesting.com
Printed in the USA
BVHW050734070222
628285BV00009B/199

9 781804 374863